6 Effective Steps To Manage Your Pcos

How Small Lifestyle Changes Make A Big Difference

Table of Contents

PCOS doesn't have to rule your life. This little gem of a book will show you exactly how small, achievable lifestyle changes make a big difference.

What you'll learn:

What is PCOS?

PCOS - polycystic ovary syndrome - is a reproductive disorder that affects up to 12% of females of age 18 to 45. If you have PCOS, you're not alone.

It was first diagnosed in 1935, but research and understanding about PCOS has come a long way since then. And you're about to uncover the very latest and most relevant lifestyle, nutrition and fitness advice.

PCOS is a genetic syndrome which means that it tends to effect females within the same family. Chances are your mother, daughters, sisters or cousins also have PCOS symptoms.

When our expert team put their heads together to develop this programme, we looked at current research from published medical journals, renowned endocrinologists and even studies by psychiatrists.

We think you're going to love what you discover here.

We've worked hard to produce a programme that we'd be proud to give our sisters, our daughters and our Mums.

This programme will help you control and even reduce four key areas which probably cause you stress and worry, and could affect your health in the long-term.

But first, let's highlight some of the medical concerns linked with a PCOS diagnosis.

PCOS And Our Modern Lifestyles

PCOS is aggravated by environmental conditions, which partly explains why symptoms are more frequently seen in first world developed countries. This can be attributed to our abundance of food, larger portions and over-reliance on junk food, and our lower levels of daily activity (but higher levels of stress and work load). In fact, our modern lifestyles are making the condition more common than ever before.

Warning Signs Of PCOS

It's common for a woman with PCOS to have a history of weight gain. Often, she'll notice a tendency to gain weight easily (very frustrating!) and upon medical examination the PCOS gene is discovered.

Other symptoms and signs of PCOS include:

- Abdominal obesity (stomach fat)

- Acne (30% of PCOS sufferers will be affected by this)

- Excess androgen levels

- Facial hair & hair in other areas (hirsutism affects 70% of PCOS sufferers)

- Scalp hair loss

- Menstrual irregularities

- Insulin resistance

- Metabolic syndrome

- Infertility

The Importance Of Insulin Resistance

Insulin resistance affects up to 50% of women with PCOS. Even lean women with PCOS are 50-70% more likely (than their non-PCOS peers) to have insulin resistance.

But what exactly is insulin resistance, and why does it matter?

Insulin resistance is particularly important to long term health, because it can lead to an increased risk of type 2 of diabetes, obesity, stroke, heart attack and cardiovascular disease.

In fact, insulin resistance is the root cause of a range of medical conditions, including metabolic syndrome, hypertensions, dyslipidemia and glucose intolerance

Women with PCOS need to be particularly aware of insulin resistance.

2% of women with PCOS will develop type 2 diabetes every single year. Within their lifetimes, 50% of women with PCOS will develop type 2 diabetes. Even if the PCOS sufferer never develops type 2 diabetes, she is still more likely to have a glucose intolerance. In fact, up to 40% of women with PCOS will have glucose intolerance (compared to only 7% of women without PCOS).

The Significance Of Metabolic Syndrome

How does metabolic syndrome show itself? In an increased risk of excess weight around the abdominal area, in elevated tri glycerides levels, elevated cholesterol levels , abnormal blood sugar levels and increased blood pressure.

Infertility & PCOS

PCOS is particularly known for causing infertility, which will actually affect 40% of women with PCOS. The most common form of infertility experience by PCOS women is an ovulatory. This means that ovulation does not take place.

Of all women who experience ovulation difficulties, a staggering 90-95% are diagnosed with PCOS. In other words, if you are experiencing any difficulties with ovulation it is likely you have PCOS, and certainly worth getting tested for.

When we look at couple infertility, 30% is due to the female having PCOS. Even when a PCOS woman isn't infertile, and is able to conceive, between 42-73% will experience a spontaneous abortion when pregnant. Sad facts, but it's important that you're aware so you can start to tackle lifestyle factors and take your PCOS under control.

Depression Disorders

As well as physical problems, PCOS sufferers are more likely to have emotional problems.

For example, over 1/3 of PCOS sufferers will have depression, 1 in 10 will have bipolar, and over 1 in 10 binge eat. The list goes on. This is exactly why we did not just look at nutrition and exercise when we put together this ground-breaking programme. We also considered mindset, stress and sleep coaching so you can manage your PCOS with a total body approach.

We mentioned earlier that the effects of PCOS could be dangerous to your long-term health.

But it's not all bad news.

By making small, sustainable dietary and lifestyle changes, women with PCOS can

- Reduce abdominal fat

- Lower testosterone levels

- Decrease hirsutism

- Improve insulin sensitivity

Sound good? Then let's get started by showing you the Six Pillars To Success. These are going to be the foundation for your management of PCOS -for life!

Introducing Your Six Pillars To Success

- Nutrition

- Water

- Exercise

- Stress

- Sleep

- Mindset

In each chapter, we'll set out lifestyle changes, and explain why they are important. We've even included activities and links to helpful PDFs.

http://www.pcoslifestylesolutions.com/Hidden/

This programme is a practical workbook for you refer to time and time again as you master your journey of recovery.

Building Block 1: Nutrition: Food Timing, Low Carb, Protein Control

Proper management of nutrition is key to the maintenance and control of PCOS.

But what does that mean?

You might feel confused or overwhelmed by the amount of conflicting information about healthy eating and diets online these days.

Nutrition is most important building block to our lifestyle solution, which is why we decided to address is first.

The three key elements we will discuss in this chapter are optimal macro nutrient combinations, portion control and meal sizes for practical everyday living and optimum timing of food.

Why are these building blocks so important? Because PCOS raises your insulin levels, causing insulin resistance which means you store glucose rather than eliminating it from your body.

Follow our guidelines and alter your insulin sensitivity, and your body will be in a better position to burn rather than store fat.

By improving your insulin sensitivity you will also reduce:

- Weight gain

- Excess hair

- Acne

- Suppressed immune system

- Increased testosterone levels

- Anxiety

Low Carbohydrates

Carbohydrates, whether complex or simple and whether from potatoes and rice or cakes and cookies, are basically sugars. Another word for this is glucose. As someone with PCOS, you have insulin resistance. We need to alter that, by reducing your intake of glucose. The easiest way to do this is to make sure that you eat proportionally fewer carbohydrates than the general population.

Let's simplify this: when you start the PCOS Lifestyle Solution programme, your carbohydrates will come from green vegetables salad vegetables and thin-skinned fruits.

Protein Intake

Another cornerstone to your PCOS-success diet is increasing your protein intake. This achieves several things: satisfying your appetite, and stabilising your blood sugars, making the use of a low carb diet more effective.

What About Fats?

The third macronutrient is fats. Unlike a lot of diet programmes, we will not be asking you to eat low fat. With the lowering of carbs, we encourage the use of fats as an alternative energy source. But remember: fats have a high calorific value, so use portion control!

Portion Control

When you join the PCOS Lifestyle Solutions programme, you'll get access to our meal planners and recipes, designed to fit the PCOS Solutions rules perfectly.

But we don't want you to wait until then, so here's an overview of portion control via some basic visual clues that you can incorporate in to your life today.

1 portion cheese and dairy– matchbox size

1 portion meat and fish – a deck of playing cards

1 portion green veg/salads – 2 fists

1 portion fats – equivalent to 10p, 1 Euro or 1 Quarter

Lowering carbohydrates, increasing protein and good portion control are standard practice with managing PCOS. But our research has uncovered one exciting element that most programmes do not incorporate: meal timings vs meal size.

Timings & Size

Eat Breakfast like a King, Lunch like a Prince and Dinner like a Pauper.

Our research has shown that, if you apply the above principle alongside our other nutrition rules, you will have the most effect PCOS nutrition solution currently known.

When designing our programme, meal planner and recipes, we took all these principles and packaged them up in a lifestyle friendly way which will help you stick with it and get genuine results for the first time ever.

It is no secret that women with PCOS have hormonal imbalances which lead to problems with losing weight. It is genuinely harder for you to lose weight! But this is not an excuse to sit on the couch feeling sorry for yourself.

With 10% of the female population currently suffering from PCOS, you are far from alone.

What this means is that 10% of women should take personal responsibility to manage their condition and not let it overwhelm them.

You have our sympathies, but we're here to support with straight talk and clear guidelines!

It's highly likely you have 'thrifty genes': inherited genes that would have made you a survivor in historical times. This makes sense; the reason you are here today is down to your ancestors' ability to survive disease famine and food shortages.

However, this puts you at a disadvantage in modern times - we rarely experience food shortages. Your body is predisposed to store food and energy in a time of famine. This might seemunfair, but there is plenty we can do about it.

Let's Take Measures To Fire Up Your Metabolism!

You may still have that predisposition to store food as fat, but you can boost your fat burning furnace. Little tricks include:

Using more hot spices in meal preparations (paprika, cayenne pepper and chilli will improve your thermogenesis)

Using cinnamon will convert sugar to energy so it will less likely be stored as fat

Acidic fruits are really helpful in reducing insulin levels. Eat half a grapefruit day (no added sugar!) to increase your insulin sensitivity

Your Appetite With PCOS

One thing you may experience is genuine hunger linked to your PCOS. This could be due to an over-production of the hormone leptin.

Leptin is a natural appetite suppressant. So isn't over-production a good thing? No - it makes you resistant to leptin's effects and you are likely to feel less full after eating.

One thing you can do is to eat more fibre-rich foods. Fibre will make you fuller for longer. Include foods with a higher fibre value at every meal.

For examples foods with higher fibre value include:

- Broccoli

- Brussels sprouts

- Artichokes

You should also drink plenty of water. This will not only help you combat water retention, but prevent you from mistaking thirst for hunger.

Did you know that your body's thirst signals are exactly the same as the signs for hunger?

Drinking a glass of water when you feel "hungry" won't do much for genuine hunger, but it will help you tune in with your body's cues and distinguish between hunger and thirst. We will have more on water later in the book.

On the topic of drinking, please try to avoid sugary drinks. They will suppress the chemicals in your body which regulate appetite. Sugary drinks fool our bodies into being hungry when we are not. A better choice would be herbal teas or even whole thin-skinned fruits.

Thyroid & PCOS

A large proportion of women with PCOS have dysfunctional thyroids. This means a slower, more sluggish metabolic rate, which of course makes it even more difficult to lose weight.

Eating oily fish such as salmon, trout, kippers, fresh tuna and mackerel will help combat thyroid dysfunction.

What About Supplements?

There are some natural supplements that could be the final piece in your effective weight loss nutrition strategy.

A good complex B vitamin is known for controlling fat metabolism and food digestion.

Chromium helps with insulin regulation and blood sugar levels. It may also assist with cholesterol levels and fat levels in your blood.

Manganese helps with absorption of good fats and stabilising blood sugar levels.

Magnesium (discussed in our chapter on sleep) is also helpful in the production of insulin.

If appetite control is an issue, zinc can help gently suppress cravings.

Later in the book we will discuss lethargy and lack of energy. Co enzyme Q-10 is helpful for energy production.

As with all supplementation, please check with your registered physician, GP or dietician. It is your responsibility to ensure that this supplementation is needed and taken at the correct levels for your needs.

Building Block 2: Water

Water is vital to your successful management of PCOS. Most people are always dehydrated. We encourage you to work up to 2 litres of water per day at first; this will rehydrated you and help you feel less hungry. All of which means a better functioning body!

As a PCOS sufferer, your hormones are out of sync and while our nutrition helps rebalance your hormones (through improving your insulin sensitivity), we can also optimise this through improved daily water intake.

Hydrated muscles are better at helping to burn fat. Dehydrated muscle is a poor fat burner. The more furnace-like your muscles, the better you'll manage your weight.

And water is an ideal carrier of hormones. This means hormones will be more effectively distributed and used throughout your body as they were intended. This is important for you because, as a PCOS sufferer, you have hormonal imbalances other women don't have to cope with.

Are you worried that improving water intake might be a challenge? Not only does the PCOS Lifestyle Solutions programme offer a variety of recipes whichflavour water (try the one below!) but we will encourage you to make small improvements in water intake over the weeks. Making this fun by having rewards and goals on your weekly and daily tasks.

Lush Lime Water

In a large class jug add:

1 large handful of ice cubes

2 limes, quartered

1 small handful of fresh mint leaves

5 strawberries, halved

Drink this water strained throughout the day

Getting enough water?

Visit http://www.pcoslifestylesolutions.com/Hidden/ for your water infographic

Building Block 3: Exercise

As fitness and nutrition experts, we know that exercise is a vital step in managing your PCOS. But it's overlooked by the majority of PCOS management programs.

We know from our own results and research that - whilst some of you may hate the idea - exercise and activity is essential for managing insulin resistance, which in turn aids weight loss.

The PCOS Lifestyle Solutions programme will introduce to you three fundamental elements of exercise in a management and sustainable manner appropriate to your lifestyle. So let's get started by introducing the three elements - and suggesting some activities.

Struggling for ideas on how to keep active?

Visit http://www.pcoslifestylesolutions.com/Hidden/ for your activity suggestion PDF

Daily Life LISS (Low Intensity Steady State)

The easiest, and (according to research) the most effective exercise for managing PCOS is daily low to moderation intensity activity, like walking.

Aim for a minimum of 30 minutes continuous walking per day

We all have busy lives, so here are a few little tricks we like to use:

1. Set your alarm for 45 minutes earlier in the morning, and walk before breakfast

2. Use your lunch hour to have a 30 minute walk, ideally to somewhere nearby which is outdoors, natural and peaceful. This will help reduce stress.

3. After work (and before getting settled at home), get your 30 minute walk in.

In addition to doing 30 minutes of exercise per day, it will greatly benefit you to incorporate more activity into your lifestyle in general.

See our infographic for fun ideas:

Resistance Training

By resistance training we mean using either your bodyweight or actual weights such as dumbbells, barbells and Kettlebells in an exercise routine. You will not get big and bulky from adopting a properly programmed resistance training routine, we promise! We recommend a rep range of between 12-15. It would be too complex to give you a workout here (without the proper support and guidelines). But what we can do is discuss the benefits of adding resistance training to your workouts:

1. Reducing the risk of developing diabetes. Weight training will improve the rate at which your body processes sugar, which in turn will reduce your risk of insulin resistance and onset diabetes. Remember, as a sufferer of PCOS you are 50% more likely to develop diabetes later in life.

2. Increased rate of fat burning. Adding a little muscle (which gives you that toned appearance) will improve fat burning throughout the day even when you are not exercising.

3. Reducing the risk of heart disease. Weight training will improve your cardiovascular health, which lowers bad cholesterol levels and blood pressure.

4. Reducing risk of osteoporosis. As a female you need to think about your bone health. Resistance training will improve bone density and thereby reduce your risk of osteoporosis post-menopause.

Stretching and Relaxation

As a counter measure to resistance training, it's important to have a regular stretching routine. It will help you get that toned, sleek look. Stretching is important for flexibility and reducing the risk of injury. It also improves the circulation of blood - which carries nutrients - to muscles and joints, so your body will function better.

Remember, this programme is all about a total body and nutrition approach to managing your PCOS. Within the PCOS Lifestyle Solutions programme, you will receive our "done for you" stretch and relaxation routine. This takes into account important factors such as your susceptibility to abdominal cramps, and focuses on improving circulation and core strength.

When embarking on an exercise programme you need to take into account the time available to you. Do not go too hard, too fast and set yourself up for failure. This ends up being demotivating. It is far better to create a five-point action plan that is totally individual to you.

For example:

"What is the one thing I can do that will improve my activity level just for today?"

It may be that you have a very busy day and cannot manage your 30 minute walk, but could manage 10 minutes of more vigorous housework. You can put that into your action plan and achieve it. You will feel far better about yourself and achieve more tomorrow if you do one small thing today - and complete it - than set yourself a bigger task that you put off or fail to achieve.

- What can I have for lunch today that will be lower in carbohydrates than my usual sandwich?

(Then prepare something.)

It's not all about food and exercise: later in this book we'll discuss stress, sleep and enjoyment of your life. If you think about you moving gently and effectively to make small positive changes, you will get there.

Visit http://www.pcoslifestylesolutions.com/Hidden/

for your stretch and relax routine

Building Block 4: Managing Stress

Stress And Fertility

In this section we are going to examine why people with PCOS are subject to more stress than those without (it's actually to do with the hormone cortisol).

Cortisol is produced in the adrenal gland, where its normal role is to control blood sugar levels, regulating your metabolism.

In someone with PCOS, testosterone levels (and everyday life stresses) mean too much cortisol. Excessive cortisol production has the opposite effect on its normal function in terms of controlling metabolism.

So you can see that you need to manage your stress, to lower your cortisol levels, so cortisol can perform its proper function within your body.

Earlier in the book we recommended that you did 30 minutes of walking outside every day. This will really go a very long way to reducing your stress levels.

Here's a tip from the team: when we need to manage stress, we try to remember that everything in life is a passing phase. Whatever situation you are in currently will be a mere nothing in a year's time. Keeping things in perspective (and keeping a gratitude journal) is one of the most effective ways of managing stress.

For example: if someone cuts you up when you are driving and you get very upset with the driver (maybe a bit of swearing and a few choice hand gestures!), who is more stressed at the situation? The driver who has disappeared, or you... the person swearing and driving with less control?

Of course there are other ways that we can manage stress too:

- Good nutrition

- Plenty of water

- Lots of sleep

- Reducing your caffeine intake

We also recommend you look into the following:

- Meditation

- Yoga

- Reducing hours on social media

- Reducing reality TV and TV news consumption

- Reading more quality fiction

- Being outside in nature

- Taking baths over showers

- Cooking from scratch, preparing whole foods

- Giving your time to others

- Making connections with old friends and family

- Being able to say "no" and put yourself first

- Make every day count

Did you know that both emotional and physical stress can actually stop women ovulating?

PCOS may already cause you to have irregular, heavy periods. Being stressed could compound the problem (and it also affects libido).

All of this of course reduces fertility. If you allow high-level stress to be persistent in your life, without taking corrective action, you are running the risk of long-term fertility.

By taking action to reduce your stress, you are improving your chances of conception.

While we are on the subject of fertility, let's talk about fertility and nutrition.

A healthy, balanced diet will help improve your chances of a healthy conception. But if conception is your goal, you also need an abundance of certain minerals in your body.

Iron

I am sure you've heard stories of women improving their iron levels by drinking Guinness. Coach Karen's own Grandmother was advised to drink half a pint of Guinness a day when she was pregnant at 39 with twin girls. But there are better ways to get more iron into your body.

Iron rich foods include:

- Eggs

- Fish

- Lean red meats

- Dark green vegetables

Zinc

Alongside iron, many women are deficient in zinc. While you can buy iron and zinc supplements, you can also supplement zinc naturally through the foods you eat.

We are fans of lean turkey, lean chicken and eggs as your main source of zinc. Another good source is almonds but we would like you to limit them to a small snack of 8 almonds per day (because of the high fat content in nuts).

Magnesium

Because we recommend supplementing with magnesium for sleep, we are less concerned about you finding food sources to supplement your magnesium levels, especially as the foods tend to be high in calories. If you prefer to find a natural source of magnesium you will find it in nuts and sunflower seeds. But please be aware of the high calories in both those food sources.

Selenium

Brazil and cashew nuts are the best natural sources of selenium. Again please using nuts sparingly.

Vitamin B-6

Really helps hormone balance and fertility. A delicious source we would approve of is watermelon.

Vitamin C

May help trigger ovulation. Good sources of vitamin C are raw fruits and vegetables, especially berries and dark green vegetables such as broccoli.

Vitamin E

Our preferred sources are oily fish and broccoli. As you can see broccoli is becoming your superfood source of fibre and vitamins!

Folic acid

Do take this in supplement form if you are intending to become pregnant (take prior to pregnancy and not just during it). Natural sources of folic acid include spinach and other dark green vegetables, citrus fruits, nuts and beans. But under no circumstances to do foods replace a folic acid supplement.

Essential fats

Found in oily fish, avocado, nuts and seeds.

We understand that it takes time and effort to create balanced, wholesome menus and recipes that not only help with weight loss but improve fertility.

That's exactly why our qualified nutritionists have created several different menus for you, using readily available ingredients, with quick to cook recipes that are all nutritionally balanced to hit your nutritional, weight loss and fertility goals.

More details of the PCOS Lifestyle Solutions programme can be found here.

And don't forget - when you join our PCOS Lifestyle Solutions programme, our mindset coaches will support you with a variety of activities that help you look at life in a new way, reducing stress so you will move forward in managing your condition and happiness.

Building Block 5: Sleep

Getting a good night's sleep is vital for you more than for someone without PCOS. Disrupted sleep or a lack of sleep will trigger changes within your metabolism will mean you will not process food as well as you should. In other words, your fat burning processes won't be as effective as we know they can be.

Although our programme lowers your carbohydrate intake to about 20 to 25% of your total calories for the day, you still need to be able to process these carbohydrate effectively. Unfortunately one of the side-effects of poor sleep patterns are increased likelihood of turning carb into unused energy. You are more likely to store the glucose as fat.

And lack of sleep is linked to raised cortisol levels. Cortisol is known as the stress hormone, and too much of it can affect your adrenal glands and lead to adrenal fatigue.

Ever noticed how, when you're in a fatigue state, you actually wake feeling as tired as when you went to asleep? You spend your day feeling exhausted, then as night-time approaches you start to feel awake! This continuous cycle of fatigue is exacerbated by an over reliance on caffeine.

Therefore our first step in improving sleep is to reduce caffeine. Our recommendation is a maximum of two coffees as a day. A strong black coffee upon waking and your second before 1 pm.

As a PCOS sufferer, it is vital to build a good sleep routine. Sleep is crucial not just for your emotional health and ability to cope with stress, but for your physical health too.

When you sleep, your body goes into repair mode by storing protein, restoring energy levels in your cells, producing growth hormones and improve your immune system.

A lack of sleep will interfere with your blood sugar levels and add to your already increased risk of diabetes, high blood pressure, obesity and heart disease.

The ideal is a minimum of 6 hours uninterrupted sleep a night (ahhh!)

Serotonin - the sleepy hormone - is produced as a result of eating starchy carb. But this programme does not allow you to eat starchy carbs in the first 12 weeks. So we recommend a large glass of warm milk alongside your magnesium supplement. Most women are magnesium deficient, and supplementing this mineral will improve your ability to sleep.

Other ways to ensure you get a decent night's sleep:

- Going to bed between 9-10 pm

- Reading a book

- Having no electronic devices in your bedroom, including your mobile phone and Facebook

- Don't use your mobile phone as an alarm clock. Buy a Lumie light alarm clock which will wake you up naturally

- Ensure your curtains are lined with blackout material so that your room can be in total darkness

- No TV in your bedroom

- Set your alarm for 6 am

- Avoid alcohol: it reduces the quality of sleep you get

You'll find our sleep diary and checklist attached. They'll both really help you improve your quality of sleep.

Visit http://www.pcoslifestylesolutions.com/Hidden/
for your sleep diary check list

Building Block 6: Mindset

The motivation for change has to come from you.

We have some incredible nutrition, exercise and mindset coaches ready to support you in taking control of your PCOS, but we cannot do the work for you.

You really have to want to change and feel better.

It has be proven that simply telling people about health risks does not make them want to change. You already know that your long-term diagnosis for serious medical conditions is not great. But a 50% risk of developing long-term diabetes might not be enough to motivate you to change. It has to come from within you.

So: do you want to feel better, look better, have better long term health, feel sexy, feminine, and confident again?

It's easy to think about starting something tomorrow or on Monday or after your holiday.

Coach Karen says: "I know my big trigger for change was sitting next my Aunt who was 6 years my senior but half my size. The very next day I took control of my nutrition and lifestyle and over the next two years lost 112lbs (50 kg)."

Your turning point might be a photograph, the desire to run a 5k, an upcoming holiday or your wish to have children.

Whatever your trigger is, write it down and place it somewhere important, learn to focus on that trigger and take action.

The fact that you're reading this book shows us that you want change. But there is a difference with wanting change and making change happen. One way to affect change today is to join PCOS Lifestyle Solutions programme. You will receive all the tools you will ever need to make positive changes in your life and condition.

In the meantime, be kind to yourself, learn to reward yourself with things other than food. It can be fun to try a new shade of lipstick, new hair colour, new style of top or new pair of shoes.

In fact, you can learn to reward yourself under the poorest of circumstances by becoming an explorer in your own life. When was the last time you took a walk around a neighbourhood and observe the surrounding views and all the quirky things? Which neighbour has a gnome in their garden, which neighbour has the best lawn, who has the most beautiful flowers?

When was the last time you went to your local museum wandering through the corridors learning something about your local or national history? Does your town have regular street entertainers so you can watch free theatre taking place in front of you? Do you ever go to a car boot sale and rummage through the boxes looking for that quirky find?

Have you ever just put your music on loud and danced for 30 minutes for no particular reason?

When was the last time you lay on the lawn and observed the shapes of clouds and created stories in your head about far off places?

These are all ways you can reward ourselves in everyday life.

There are even things about domestic life that can be a pleasure, rather than a chore! For example, a new coat of paint to freshen a room up gives a feeling of achievement and pleasure that you'll miss from simply vacuuming and cleaning it.

Coach Karen has already told you that it took her two years to lose 112 lbs (50kg). When she started that journey, she never thought it would take that long. "If I had, I might have given up," she says. "What helped me was living in the now, achieving for the day, keeping my trigger in mind, and having a definite non-food reward system in place.""

When you join PCOS Lifestyle Solutions, you'll get access to a group of coaches who all want you to be successful.

But this is not a 100 metre sprint.

The programme is called Lifestyle Solutions for a reason: we know what will get you to your goals and ultimately change your life:

- small steps

- being consistent every day

- being persistent

- having reward systems

- great support

- doing the best type of exercise

- eating the correct types of food at the right times of the day

During your first 12 weeks of the PCOS Lifestyle Solutions programme you will be given fun weekly goals. These will not always be nutrition or exercise related. Sometimes they focus on putting yourself first and looking after yourself.

To give you a taster of the sort of activities we are talking about, we have included a downloadable PDF of your daily diary. It is an incredible self-awareness and coaching tool which will help you examine the quality of each day that you live, rather than making it through to every evening exhausted and drained. Questions like "what did I enjoy most about my day?" will give you time to genuinely reflect on making the most of your day. It's often the small pleasures in life which give us our reason for being.

Visit http://www.pcoslifestylesolutions.com/Hidden/ for your daily diary

Conclusion

We hope that our introductory guide to the six pillars of success have given you hope - and clarity - that PCOS is manageable. With the very best support, guidance and advice, you can make massive changes to your future health, happiness, body and weight.

We have shown you that following a low carb nutrition programme along with portion control can dramatically improve your insulin sensitivity.

In the chapter on water, we gave you a link to help you achieve drinking two litres of water a day, and guidelines in reducing caffeine, sugary drinks. We even added a natural, great tasting recipe.

We then took you through the importance of daily activity in helping reduce stress and boosting your metabolism and insulin sensitivity.

We went on to discuss the potential risk of modern lifestyle stress, with the increased production of cortisol affecting your metabolism. We showed you how you can improve your ability to burn fat and use calories more effectively by reducing stress.

The final chapter on mindset encapsulates our whole body approach. The full PCOS Lifestyle Solutions programme has weekly coaching activities to help you frame positive experiences to be happier, healthier and leaner.

A Final Note From The PCOS Lifestyle Solutions Coaches

Congratulations on taking a huge step towards a healthier future, and thank you for purchasing this book. We'd love to hear your reviews, questions and feedback. And we hope to see you on our 12 week Specialist Programme.

Visit www.pcoslifestylesolutions for our early bird special offer

Copyright © 2015

Karen Nadkarni Ruffle

Ben Knight

Kelly West

ISBN-10: 1517394031
ISBN-13: 978-1517394035

www.ingramcontent.com/pod-product-compliance
Lightning Source LLC
Chambersburg PA
CBHW072022290526
45787CB00013B/1739